DEALING WITH ANXIETY DEPRESSION PTSD OR ALL THREE

Author Jessica D Moore
Editor B Houston

Dedicated to all who go through anxiety, depression, and PTSD (Post Traumatic Stress Disorder), without people understanding these things and being there to help you. It is also for those who have been through any of these and came out of it. To all my family and friends who are going through these or have been through these. EVERYONE REMEMBER KEEP YOUR HEAD UP AND YOU GOT THIS!

Copyright©2020 by Jessica D Moore
All rights reserved. No part of this book may be reproduced or used in any manner without written permission of the copyright owner except for the use of quotations in a book review.

ANXIETY

      Mental health is an especially important thing to all humans whether young or old and no matter what race. Anxiety, depression, and PTSD (Post Traumatic Stress Disorder) are a few of the top mental illnesses that exist in our society. When a person has (anxiety, depression, or PTSD) these things, many times you are not able to tell by just looking at them. Usually a person that has these illnesses will be the main one making everyone laugh and find themselves crying when they are by themselves. If you know a person going through any form of mental illness, take a moment of your day to check in on them. Nine out of ten times if they come to you about the problems they are facing, take a second to listen and try not to judge or be too hard on them. Judging them could cause them to spiral even more out of control and shut down. If a person happens to tell you that they have anxiety, depression, or PTSD, try not to think of them as crazy or make them feel embarrassed or ashamed that they have it. Doing these things to people that have illnesses like these will make them feel less than a person. Remember sometimes all it takes it one person being there for another one, whether family, friend, or a newfound friend.

      This is for those that may not understand what anxiety, depression, and PTSD is. I plan to break it down in a way that can hopefully be understood by most. But before I get into everything and give a break it down, I want to start with a little note by saying that a person can have PTSD even if they have never been in the military. I will get more in depth with this in another chapter. But let us talk about how anxiety is a real thing and how when you are going through it, you will feel like the world is smothering you. With a person feeling smothered, you tend to find yourself gasping for air at a very rapidly pace. The more you feel the need to gasp for air, the more you find yourself focusing on what caused you to have the anxiety attack. The more a person focuses on the reason behind what is causing the anxiety attack, the more the person will find themselves becoming more anxious.

      There are many things that can trigger an anxiety attack. Stress is one of the largest causes of a lot of anxiety attacks that people experience. The stress could come from work, friends, marriages, and a variety of other things. While a certain amount of stress can be good for our lives, an abundance of stress is very harmful. Stress can even be so harmful that it can be a cause of death. Most people think that when a person is having an anxiety attack but is not hyperventilating that they could be faking it. What many people do not realize is that everyone experiences anxiety attacks differently. Anxiety can also come at some of the weirdest times. For example, when the day came to leave to go on my vacation, I started to have an anxiety attack in the form of freaking out and being very nauseated. The first time I took a vacation where I was flying on a plane, I blacked out while being on the plane.

      That incident on the plane happened when I was younger, but as I got older, I would actually throw up before boarding a plane, usually on the car ride to the airport. Now that I am older, I have figured out ways that I can calm myself down before it happens. One of the main ways of controlling my anxiety is by taking a deep breath in through my nose, and slowly exhaling out from my mouth. Secondly, I try to focus all my thoughts to a place that brings me peace. I try to focus on how much I would enjoy myself if I were at these places. For example, I will picture myself on a beach with white sand and clear blue water. I imagine seeing the water crashing up on the beach, which helps bring a calming spirit over me.

      What a lot of people fail to realize is that most people suffer with anxiety from a young age. However, I believe the weirdest part is that many people do not realize is that most people end up with anxiety as they become older. The problem with having anxiety as you get older is that there is stress added to our lives by way of having more responsibilities. I know most of my anxiety comes from me growing, but I have always been a worry wart type of person. While growing up as a youth, some of the things I used to worry about is how I look from other people eyes for not having the top brand name clothes, or not having my hair done in the popular styles that people sported.

    Now a days we live in a society where a lot of people have anxiety, and most of us that suffer through this are embarrassed to get help. The most critical first step that a person dealing with anxiety should do is get help with their anxiety from a qualified professional medical person (doctor, counselor, or psychiatrist). When it comes to our health in general, it should be of upmost importance since our mental health is a large part of being healthy. Your mental health is precious, and I view it as being the new wealth. I mean if you do not have your mental health, you cannot achieve much. There are many levels to dealing and coping with anxiety. Sometimes anxiety can be calmed by just talking to someone all the way up to even taking medications. If you happen to know someone that is going through anxiety, being there for them can sometimes make all the difference. Sometimes all a person needs are listening ears to get through the day. Yes, I know everyone goes through things at times, but if we took the time to listen to one another, we might just find ourselves dealing less with mental health related issues.

    A lot of kids get anxiety from having to take test in schools and then the other test that the states get to make sure they are learning in their classes. People that take test get anxiety whether they study or not. It is just the fact that knowing that you must remember everything you either learned in that week or over a few weeks and hope that you can answer the questions correctly. Some kids are nervous at taking test because they may have something at stake. Basically, if they are an athlete, they know that the test may be most of the grade and if they do not pass it and fail, they will get kicked off the team. Or it could even mean that they are taking a test to get into the college of their dreams and need a certain score to get in. Then there is just those who seem to be nervous when they must take a test.

    Another part of the puzzle when it comes to mental health that we are missing is that people these days focus too much on social media, and we have less of a human connection with others. Less human connection tends to have people in their heads wondering what other people think of them, or if they even care or love them. When it comes to social media, we have become more concerned with being liked by other people and seeking what they have, rather than being ourselves. Trying to be like others and live the way they do can add more stress into your life, which can cause you to become anxious. Yes, sometimes being yourself will cause anxiety, but I personally would rather have anxiety being myself than to have it while trying to be someone I am not. It is always better to be unique and be yourself. Most of us fail to realize that a lot of people on social media are portraying an image that they have all this stuff, when in reality many of them do not have much of what they're pretending to have. In all cases but especially this case make sure you love yourself first and the hardest.

    There are people that get anxiety from having to bring who they love home to meet their family. Basically it could be for many reasons like example, it could be they are dating someone of a different race that their parents will not approve of, the family may not think anyone is good enough to date their family member, it could be because they are not of the same religion, the fact of the person coming from the same kind of background, and lastly when you bring someone of the same sex home. A lot of time it becomes hard for people that are homosexual to come out to people in their schools, jobs, communities, and among their friends.

That means that people can get anxiety from falling in love with someone they never expected, because they may get rejected and cast out of their loved ones lives for loving who they love. We all need to remember that just because our loved one may not be with who we want them to be with, we need to remember that they are human and still need our love. I mean if the person that they love is harmless, it should not matter to their loved ones. Anxiety over stuff like this should not exist it should be whoever they are happy being with. It does not mean that you must like the person they are with but at least love the person for respecting you enough to let you know who they love.

     Parents can give their kids anxiety and not even realize it because while their choices may make the parent happy it can give the child stress and cause anxiety. For example if you decide that you want to be with the same sex after your child gets to a certain age then it could put them in a situation where they get bullied because they do not have a mommy and a daddy but either two moms or two dads. So, the child or children will get anxiety having to go to school knowing that they will get bullied for their parent's choices. What a parent might not realize is that kids will be mean to other kids more than ever. A lot of them being mean to other kids and giving them anxiety is because of what they are taught at home on the daily basis.

     When a parent have a child and end up without the other parent whether it is due to death, the parents do not get along, or they do not want the child, make sure whoever you bring into your children's life that they will treat them just like their own, and make sure not to treat the person you are with better than your kids that you made. This can give them anxiety because they will feel alone in this big world that we are in. For example if your spouse is not around and you treat your children with all the care in the world, but when your spouse walk in you cater to them and make your children clean up behind your spouse and let your spouse lounge around all day that is a way for your children to get anxiety attacks knowing that they have to be around someone who you treat better than them. Parents need to remember that it is okay to have your child help around the house doing chores, but they should not have to do them alone, because they are not the only ones making the mess around the house.

     Anxiety can come in many different forms. In my case, I often find myself worrying about things I cannot control in life. I believe most of my anxiety comes from something that is common in everyone's lives, change. No matter how much we do not want certain things to change, change is always happening whether for the better or worse. However, if we want to make it to our dreams in life, we must endure change. Even just writing about how anxiety can be caused by change makes me want to have an anxiety attack. However, I also know if I do not invite change into my life, I will not get anywhere near where I want to be. I know that change can be scary and a big cause of anxiety. Much of this is because we all have a fear of the unknown. For example, you do not know what will happen if you hang out with a person that you have a crush on. If you do not take that leap of faith to find out, you will never know if you and the person could have been more. However, if you do take that leap, will the person you have feelings for make you realize you do not like them no more than a friend? It can be a scary situation due to the unknown that comes along with it. Change can also trigger anxiety because of not knowing one way or another how things will turn out. Anxiety can also coincide with change if it is something that you do not want to do, or something that seems very scary to you.

     Another way some people can get anxiety is losing someone that is very close to you. These people are not only limited to but can include a mother, father, sister, aunt, brother, uncle, grandmother, grandfather, or friend. Other factors can depend on how a person that is close to you dies, and how close you were to them before they transitioned. When my mom died of cancer, I was 19 years old. So, when I had one symptom that my mom had, I would freak out and think that I had cancer. It is amazing how our brains can make us feel anxious about something like this, and it is all because of one symptom and the fact that we were related to someone that died from a disease that includes a symptom we may have had. I mean when you lose someone close to you, it may freak you out because they may have done a lot of things for you in your life. Now you find yourself in a situation where you must figure out how to do so many things on your own. You could also deal with anxiety from having things change from not having that extra person around. It may freak you out even more so because you do not have that person there anymore to talk to and hold a conversation. Fear and worry can give us a lot of anxiety.

      Anxiety can also come from having a disease or something that can cause you to die prematurely. You might find yourself having an anxiety attack for the fact of knowing if you do anything wrong, you could lose your life. Anxiety may exist for someone that may have a disease like diabetes and must watch everything that they eat, along with hoping that their sugar does not spike too high or drop too low. Then there are people who may have body parts that are not functioning correctly. They are hoping that the medication that they are given, or a surgical procedure will help keep them alive longer. This is another example of how you may never know that a person has anxiety. I mean there are people who have anxiety because they must get shots every day to live or find themselves staying in a hospital for months at a time. Some people will even have anxiety because they know they have a long road ahead of them in order to get their health in a better shape. When people have medical problems, we never know how many of them may be going it alone and be super nervous about it. For some, trying to achieve the wealth of mental health or their health in general is hard.

      Then there are the people who are anxious because they have a loved one going through something medically or life changing. It is stressing them out, which also makes us stress out as well. When a person loves someone enough, when they see their loved ones going through something difficult, it will stress them out also. They can stress until they potentially end up having an anxiety attack. For example, if a parent must see their baby go into surgery or get a biopsy to make sure that their health is okay, this will obviously stress the parents and may cause an anxiety attack. They always say that there is no love like a parent's love. Parents love hard for their kids, and a lot of times they may have anxiety because they want their kids to have a great life. Parents may worry if they are doing the right things to make sure their kids are on the right path towards success and not on a path towards getting in trouble. I mean no parent wants to see their kids go down the wrong path such as joining a gang, stealing, or killing. Since parents come under a lot of stress, they tend to have anxiety attacks over worrying about their kids being okay every second of everyday.

      Another thing that may cause a person to develop anxiety is being married to someone who they are around all the time. A lot of times people think that just because you love someone that they will not have things about them that will cause you to feel anxious. They may be romantic and loving towards you, and they may never raise their voice or get upset. However, a marriage can change quite a bit as time goes on. A lot of times a person can be anxious not knowing how to live with someone other than the family that they grew up with, and not knowing what someone else living ways are can increase anxiety levels. Often, two people may find that they can get along simply fine without them living together. There may be a little stress every now and then, but when you see them every day and have a routine set up, it can change everything you are used to doing. The stress of changing your routine and trying to compromise with a person to make things work can bring a lot of stress in your life, which in turn can cause an anxiety attack. Many people do not realize that some people fake being the true person they are until they are super comfortable with the person, which ultimately means that a lot of times people will get someone who is really nice and sweet in the start. Then you may find later down the line that the person may turn out to be mean and rude. Also, with marriage, you get the other person's debt and bills, which can cause a lot of stress and can turn into and cause anxiety attacks.

     Another way people end up having anxiety attacks is having to worry about if they will make enough money to pay their bills. Some people may have to work more than one job just to make ends meet and to be able to keep a roof over their head and food on their table. With the person being under so much stress they tend to have and anxiety attack because they may not have anyone else to turn to for help. The person that is struggling may have an anxiety attack worrying about where their next meal and check is coming from. In the back of the persons mind will be the thought of if they do not get money, they will end up homeless and, on the streets, begging for money.

     Kids that are orphans tend to have anxiety growing up and not really having a family. They get bullied by other kids especially when they find out that they do not have a family like everyone else. These kids end up having an anxiety attack because they do not get to have a lot of the finer things in life, it is basically hand me downs or cheap clothes. These kids have anxiety attacks when they are given group projects that they work on outside of the school. Many kids will talk about them when they figure out that they do not really have a loving family waiting for them at home. Which the child now has the fear that the other student is going to go back to school and tell everyone about their situation. These kids also must deal with the anxiety of whether they will ever be adopted.

     Children must deal with the fact that sometimes in order to be popular are liked at school you must do some crazy things. Kids are under the pressure of their peers which can cause them a lot of anxiety. For example, if the popular kids are illegally drinking the one that wants to fit in will drink even though they really do not want to. This could cause them a lot of anxiety because they know at home they will get in trouble, but if they do not do it then they will not be part of the in crowd. Sometimes as parents we forget how hard it is to fit in with the people around us and just fuss about everything that kids do wrong that will cause them to have anxiety. We as adults sometimes even have anxiety from not fitting in at our jobs or our communities.

     Anxiety can come from parents comparing their kids to one another. This can even happen as they get older and choose their career paths. The parents may not like the fact that one child is in a field that does not pay a lot of money, so they criticize them in turn causing them to have an anxiety attack. I mean if the adult child is happy in their career choice the parent should be happy. But comparing the jobs of adult kids can cause anxiety attacks if you hear it enough from a parent. Parents need to realize that not everyone is meant to have top paying jobs, that sometimes people follow their dreams. I mean if they are not living with you and they are paying their own bills, the parents should be happy.

     Anxiety can come from either being abused or watching their loved ones be abused. If they are being abused every time, they see the person that is abusing them they will start to have an anxiety attack. But if they are watching a parent get abused, they can have an anxiety attack every time they see it happen to their parent. A lot of times if the parent is not careful the child could end up in the same kind of relationship because they are used to being around that kind of relationship. Which in turn can cause them a lot of anxiety because they are getting abused on the daily. Anxiety will be a constant because they do not know if they will get through the next abuse alive and may refuse to leave because of fear or they think that they love the person that is abusing them.

Anxiety in adults sometimes come from people looking down on them for where they decided to live. Maybe it is because it is not in the fancy part of town. It could be because they do not have a big house like someone else. Basically, it is when other adults do not approve of where the other person stay. It could be because they know or think the person makes good money and should have better. What other adults may not realize is that some people would rather keep the simple things and spend money on the necessity. Meaning they would rather spend money on food and things needed and save the rest in case of an emergency, or for when they retire, they will have extra cash. Because you get more money and keep spending more of it, the longer the person will either stay in debt, become into debt, or live paycheck to paycheck.

A lot of times workaholics will have anxiety because they are always working and never have fun. They tend to have attacks if they are not working because they think that they will lose a lot of money. Workaholics tend to forget about the world around them and that you sometimes must stop relax and enjoy the things of the world. Anxiety comes from working so hard or too little and not knowing how to find a healthy balance between the two. The best thing to do is figure out if you do anything fun or do too many fun things and barely have funds to afford your activities.

Anxiety attacks can come from some of the weirdest things like boxing all your feelings up and pushing them down inside and not letting them out. Sometimes I know it is easier to say what is on your mind to some people, but some people really push how they feel inside down. For example, when you love someone but do not want to ruin your friendship, you push those feelings down in your gut and try to ignore them. This can even go for people who are friends that are secretly in love with their friend. In other words, it is easier to keep the person in your life as a friend then to not have that person in their life.

Another aspect of anxiety is career and work. A person can get anxious when they are looking for new jobs or moving from a location that they are remarkably familiar with. When you are looking for a new job, the stress behind wondering if the jobs you are applying for will reject or invite you to interview with them can trigger an anxiety attack. A person can also find themselves being anxious if they are let go from a job they enjoy because of someone else's mistakes. Sometimes it becomes crazy knowing that the job you are in now sucks, but because of anxiety, we tend to stay at that job to avoid change and the unknown. Furthermore, sometimes with getting a new job comes the task of having to move to a new location whether it is across town, in a different city, or even in a new state or country. The idea of moving just on its own is stressful. Trying to decide what to take with you when you move, what to get rid of, and what things you can or cannot take with you adds stress. I mean it even comes down to trying to organize things into boxes so that when you get to the new place you can find everything right off. All of this can be stressful, which can lead to anxiety.

Children tend to get anxiety from playing video games that are not for their age groups. For example, if you buy a child in elementary a game that is rated mature. Playing video games where it is very graphic in detail and codon a lot of fighting where you see the blood coming out. When kids start having to compete against others online and they start losing a lot, or they cannot get passed levels it starts to stress them out to the point of having anxiety. Children a lot of times will get a lot of anxiety from not being able to play these games all the time and will send them into an anxiety attack because they think that the world revolves around it. Another instance is they play to many shooting games where they have to hunt and kill other players inside or around houses, with the other players jumping out at them, can cause an anxiety attack at night in the home, with them thinking someone is waiting around the corner for them and is going to kill them. Video games that are played above their age limit online, and playing with adults, can scare them or give them an anxiety attack, because you will have some adults that will make them feel like they know where the child lives. The adults online will even say mean and hurtful things, which can in turn cause anxiety attacks. The other thing that might give them anxiety attacks are the fact of adults insulting the kids or their parents.

    Anxiety with me comes from the unknown. What I mean is if I have people in my life a lot of times, I am scared to say anything to them that may hurt their feelings, which means it stays buttoned up inside me, so they do not hurt. It has been so many times that people that I genuinely care about hurt me, but instead of saying anything in the moment or at all I keep it to myself. Which truly means I am the only one that is getting hurt. Because at the end of the day my friends and family will tell me that I hurt them, which in turns will stress me out and make me have bad anxiety attacks. The reasoning behind this is I do not want them to hurt because of me and now I must find a way to fix the problem. Sometimes the anxiety attack can come from the fact of me trying to do a simple gesture and they feel like I am being mean or rude.

    Anxiety for me also comes from thinking what if I do all the hard work it takes to make a book or get a promotion, but in the end, I get rejected. I know most people say you should not care what other people think of you, but at the end of the day we all care to a certain extent. I mean I get anxiety thinking what if this book hurts anyone's feelings. I know most people would be like who cares, I do because I know what it is like to be hurt.

    I know one of my biggest anxiety attacks that I had recently, was since covid-19 started no one is allowed in a lot of places together. Well, we all know that covid-19 will give many anxiety attacks not knowing if you will catch it and watching so many people you know get it or even die from the illness. But my anxiety attack came from me having to have surgery, I could not take my medications (my anxiety pill), then no one was allowed in the building with me while I was waiting to have the procedure. I mean when you are laying in the prep area alone with no one to keep your mind occupied, you tend to go through everything bad that can happen in the operation room. For me to get through this I had to think of the health benefits after, and how my friends on the outside were rooting for me on the other side. And then of course they gave me anxiety medication through intravenous therapy (iv) I knew everything would be simply fine. Sometimes the best thing to do in certain situations is stay calm and not become anxious and look at all the good that will come out of it.

    As you may be able to see, stress plays a major role in people having anxiety attacks. That is why if you feel yourself getting overwhelmed with your life, stop and take a break. Whatever is going on that is causing you stress, just come back to it later after you relax. I say this because as I have found out from my own experience, a lot of times when we experience anxiety, it often comes from us trying to control things we have no control over. So, in my words, you must let go and let things happen as they may. The main thing you need to always remember is when you are having an anxiety attack, slow your breathing and try to focus on something that gives you happy thoughts and not what is causing the attack. Also remember that you are never alone when it comes to dealing with anxiety. There are always other people that go through having anxiety attacks even though they may be having their attacks for different reasons. But mainly remember that you have a least one person that will help you get through it.

DEPRESSION

Many people deal with depression and are embarrassed to admit to it for the fear of being called crazy. The main thing that people go through with depression is feeling sad and like life appears for everyone around you as being incredibly happy. Another way to think of what someone feels when they are depressed is like having the sunshine for everyone, while your days are dark from the time you wake up till the time you go to bed. Depression is like a battle within yourself every second of everyday, and that is a battle that is not an easy one to win.

Be mindful of what you tell and do to others around you. I say this because you never know what the people around you are going through, nor do you know what effect that you have on that person maintaining their life. What I mean by this is when you talk about how a person looks, which could be anything from the physical to the type of clothes a person wear. It could also be the way a person chooses to wear their hair, or if a person happens to wear glasses. Some people fail to realize that everyone is not made the same, and not everyone has as much money as someone else. A lot of times when a person hears awful things about themselves from others enough times, they start to believe it. This in turn can cause the person to be sad and think of themselves in a negative way regardless of what people who may think that they are amazing think. That person will likely have the perception that they are a horrible looking person. With people putting all these thoughts into a person's head can cause people to have depression with the thoughts of never being pretty or handsome enough for anyone to love.

A person that is depressed will often fight with themselves about many things. This can include things such as whether they should hang out with their friends or stay home and sleep in comfort. The depression that a person experiences usually sides with everything that will strip you of happiness by finding excuses of why you cannot do it. For example, if a person asks you out on a date, you might tell the person yes in the moment, but when it gets close to going out, you might think of something like they only asked me out because they feel sorry for me. So generally, with thinking this thought with depression, you can talk yourself out of going on the date. The next step is usually to find a lie to make sure that you do not hurt the other person when you tell them that you cannot go out on a date with them. You may even fight with yourself over treating yourself to something you may really want. This can happen because a lot of times people that are depressed would rather say that they have enough with what they already have.

Another thing about depression is that you have really bad thoughts most of the time. I personally refer to it as being in a bad headspace. For example, you know a lot of people that have struggled with depression have likely thought of ways to end their lives. Most people may not even realize that a depressed person is thinking this, and if they do find out, they will often tell them that by thinking this way they are selfish. However, the person is thinking of ways to end it all to get rid of all their pain and sadness. So, if you know someone that deals with depression, try to be there for them and encourage them to get help from a medical professional. Sometimes if you have a really good friend that will stick by you through it all and show you how you are better than the thoughts you are having in your head, they are a true friend. With depression having a really genuine friend next to you goes a long way.

What most people do not realize is that when a person has depression, and are trying to get help with battling it by going to counseling or taking medications, the person that is fighting the depression is strong and amazing. Think about it, they are strong because they are facing the world with thoughts of harming themselves, as well as trying to stay happy and live life. Many people do not realize that people with depression may be thinking of killing themselves at this moment and someone that was rude them is what probably what got them to that point. A person can help in causing someone with depression end it with saying stuff like "no one cares about your day", or by being mean to them for no reason at all. I was always told to smile because you never know whose day you will light up verses frowning and giving a mean look to someone. Think of it as smiling can make a person's day brighter, or it can help a person dealing with depression live to see another day. I know that some of the meanest people are customers complaining about the smallest things. You can make the person who is trying to do their job ten times harder by constantly complaining. So, try being a friendlier person towards them while they are doing their job verses being mean to them. Kindness goes an exceptionally long way when a person is dealing with depression.

      If you are dealing with depression, do everything you can to not give up on the fight. I know from experience that you can make it through the all the worst days that you have, are going to have in the future, and have been through already. The thing is that when dealing with depression and making the decision to fight against it, remember to never give up when the fighting gets tough. You must just keep pushing through the pain. If you get down, remember to pick yourself up and keep fighting. Depression is not an easy path to fight but giving up your life is not the answer either. Like a good person I know once told me; when you have the thoughts of wanting to end your life, think of how selfish you are being to those that love you. Most of all, think about the things you will be leaving behind; the things you really love doing. For example, some of the things you may miss if you take your life are things such as, watching football, watching movies, eating your favorite foods, and more things that you enjoy doing while living. I was also taught that you must focus on the people that you know love you. Whether it be a family member or friend, and sometimes it can even be a co-worker who you never payed attention to how they treat you. What keeps me from wanting to harm myself and ending it all is thinking of people like my nephews (who constantly remind me of how much they love me), my godchildren (whose faces light up when I am around), and many other people that I enjoy being around. Knowing that these people would miss me being here is enough for me to keep persevering in this life I have been given.

      I mean listening to what my positive true friends say when they tell me that I help them get through some of their hardest times. Sometimes it just takes me being there for them when one of their family members are going through surgery, or when they have some uncomfortable tension with people around them, and you need someone that can lighten the mood; I am that person. So sometimes when you feel the need to end it all, you should think of how much the people around you actually count on you, as well as how some people might be ready to give up on some things they're facing in their lives. With my battle with depression, helping others is what helps me get out of having bad thoughts. With depression, if you do other things to stay busy like working or journaling in a diary, it can keep you from thinking so hard on what is making you depressed. If you keep your mind occupied, you tend to be better off. When you find yourself being depressed, it is better to try to keep yourself busy, then to try to sleep.

      Depression can be defeated by a person finding something that can be of interest to them, and then using it to get through the tough times. I know with me personally, the things that helped me to get through depression were starting my own blog, as well as taking up teaching myself how to draw and paint. These new interests are what ended up leading me here to write a book. I felt that if I wrote a book on my experience with anxiety and depression, I could help someone else that is going through the same thing. The hope I have is to inspire others to keep their life and find something that inspires them to change their lives. Just because a person deals with depression does not mean that they are not able to come out of it. I believe that a person can still have it and inspire others. Inspiring others with depression can help the person you are helping, as well as yourself. The reasoning behind this is that a lot of times we feel good from helping others, as well as helping us to keep our minds occupied.

   There are many ways to occupy your mind, but you also have to learn ways to be able to shut your mind down at the end of the night. What I mean is a lot of times when you are dealing with depression, your mind will not shut off due to the fact of thinking of ways to inspire other people. However, your mind is mainly thinking of the ways that you can end your life. Some of the worst ways you cannot get your mind to shut off is when you start thinking of all the mean things people have said or done to you. You have to realize that nine out of ten times when they are bullying you or being rude, the reasoning behind it is that they are going through abuse or depression, and they do not know how to deal with it effectively. Thus, they take it out on others.

   Depression can be like a bad cryptic mind game that you must be strong-minded to understand and make it out of. Sometimes you may have depression to the point that you will not make it out dealing with it, rather you will have to learn how to fight with it daily. Even if this turns out to be the case for your life, make sure you never give up. Depression in teens and younger kids can happen frequently because they get bullied a lot, and there is so much pressure on them to do things that only adults should be doing. Depression can come from a parent putting too much pressure on their kids to do well in school. I get it, you want the kids to do better and achieve their goals, but sometimes you must let a kid be a kid. Parents sometimes get frustrated with kids when they are dealing with depression because they are unruly from the fact that they do not always know how to deal with their depression. They may even not understand what depression is. If you know a parent that has a kid that may be dealing with this and the parent seems to be getting frustrated, please try to give the parent a break by either babysitting the child, or getting someone to babysit so you can take the parent out to let them breathe for a bit. When a child has depression, sometimes it is best for both the parent and child to first find a way to calm down. Going for a walk in the park or doing something fun can help with this. Once the parent and child are calm, they need to have a discussion without judgment about why their child is feeling down and sad. If you are a parent that feels you cannot listen to your child judgment free, then bring them to see a professional. Adults have to keep in mind that just like you have feelings, so do kids, and it does not matter what age they start having depression, be there.

   Depression can stem from some very simple things that we have in our lives. Depression, just like anxiety can come from change happening. An example of this is when you have a bad trait or habit that you know you need to change, but you either do not know where to start, or you feel like you are not going anywhere no matter how hard you try. I mean one thing I have been trying to work on that gives me depression, along with my anxiety is not letting my walls all the way down, or being able to control my feelings as much as I like. Also, the fact of not letting my emotions lead me into things I know are not right. Depression can come when you think you have found your mate, but they turn out to be completely opposite, or they turn out to be a better friend than a companion. I mean some people would say that they would rather have a person they fell for to be a friend than not to have them at all.

Depression can also have you holding onto people that you know need to be out of your life. People with depression also need to learn the fact that if you let someone go and they come back, they are yours to keep. However, if you let them go and they do not come back, they were never yours. I used to get told a lot of times that some people are only meant to be in your life for a season, not a lifetime. But when you have depression to the point where you do not let people go, you tend to end up having fake friends in your life. For a person not battling depression, letting go of someone is hard, however when you have depression in your life, it can be extremely hard to let go. You tend to feel this way because you feel like if you let them go, you are making a big mistake, which in turn can cause a lot more problems for you. As one person once told me before, if someone wants to leave, let them because that means they no longer want to be there. Trying to keep a person that no longer wants to be in your life will have you constantly sucking up to them in order to keep them. It is not worth it when they will probably still end up leaving. So, a person with depression that is holding onto someone will often do this as a way of asking for help. However, at the same time it will drain them of a lot of their happiness and peace. Those of us that battle depression feel as if we need people in order to feel like we are complete, and we often do not realize that we do not need other people in order to be a complete person. Being a person with depression will sometimes have you forgetting that you are complete with or without another person.

A person with depression can sometimes feel like they need to be helping someone or need someone to need them in order to feel like they're doing something to help make a mark in the world. When having depression, sometimes helping others can make people with depression forget about what they are going through in their own lives. Sometimes when you have depression, forgetting about your own problems to help others makes you feel a lot of better. Even if it is for a moment, it is better than being depressed every moment of your day. When you stop and think about it, a lot of times people who are depressed do not get to enjoy any good moments for the sake of all the bad thoughts that are going through their heads regularly. For example, they may be thinking of ways to kill themselves such as if they're driving over a bridge or overpass, they may think of how letting go of the wheel will send them over the edge to end it all. The good thing is that a lot of times people will not act on these kinds of thoughts, especially if they have already sought professional help.

Since we are all different people, we all deal with depression differently. Usually if a person is going to commit suicide, they will just do it without anyone finding out till the deed is done. But what other people must realize is that a lot of the time, the people that are dealing with this kind of depression will be asking for help in the strangest ways. For example, if you have a person that is normally quiet or follow the rules and now you notice that they are being super loud and breaking the rules, it usually means they are trying to seek attention. This usually is a cry for help because they are depressed. Not all people who change like this are looking for help with depression. It could also be them dealing with abuse at home as well, or that they are finally gaining their freedom.

Another type of way a person may get depression is by being abused, or finding out someone that you are close to has been abused in some way by someone else that you may know. The reason a person can get depression from finding out someone close to them has been abused is because there is nothing that you can do to make the abused person feel better. You have a desire to help, or to change the past so it does not happen at all. Depression also comes from feeling helpless in these kinds of situations. If you do not get any kind of help with dealing with this kind of depression, it can lead to being angry a lot, as well as pushing a lot of people away because you feel like everyone is going to end up knowing or doing the same things. With this type of depression, people tend to be more embarrassed than anything. Going through this situation it is not something to be ashamed of, and a lot of times it is better if you speak out about it. You never know who you are helping get out of their situation by you making it out of yours.

    People will never understand that people with depression will seem normal except for a few signs, like not having self-esteem, smiling all the time, cheering everyone else up, giving all of them for someone else's happiness, etc. No, I am not saying everyone that does this has to have depression, but most of the people that do this does. I mean someone like me who has a big heart does this, while I am hurting on the inside on the outside no one would ever know. I mean even when I work, I fight the heart ache and work till my job is done even when my body may be aching, along with my heart. People never realize that a person with depression has to fight extra hard to make sure that no matter how down and worthless they feel they need to get up and continue normal easy things like eat or go to work. If you let a person that has depression just sit around and think without them having hobbies a lot of times, they end up thinking of all the things they have done wrong, or even worse things that people have done wrong to them that they let them get away with and know they blame themselves for. As a person who struggle with mental illness everyday it is not a day that goes by that I do not feel like giving up everything and just sleep away this life. But I know that will not help me achieve any of my dreams like writing this book to help people become aware of how it feels to live with these different mental illnesses.

    Some people with depression look for pity, I do not I want to be seen normal as possible. For example, I deal with health issues besides my mental health, but I would rather struggle through it and get better than to be pitied. I mean that fact of the matter is I may have to work harder at everything I do, but at least I know that at the end of the day it was my hard work and not someone feeling sorry for me that help me make it to where I want to be. I also know that there are times when I do need help to get things done, to which I will ask for help. But because I must work harder than others, I also know that I must sometimes take my pride out of it and lend a hand or ask for one.

    I think one of the hardest things I have had to do since being diagnosed with these mental illnesses is telling my boss at work if I start acting weird, to let me know because my doctor put me on a medication to try to calm down some of the sadness. The reason it is so embarrassing because when I first started out, I was getting tried on so many different medications to see what would work. For example, I had a medication that was supposed to help me be alert and focused, but instead it turned out that it made me real sleepy and by me wanting to make sure that I could get home properly, I had to leave work early. That is not telling anyone that decides to get medication to help with their mental illness that this will happen, some people get the first pill, and it works for them.

    When it comes down to depression, a lot of people will not talk about it for the sake of feeling embarrassed or crazy if people know that they deal with it. I have even heard of instances of people losing their jobs because people find out about their battle with depression. People with depression will often quit everything, including their job, because dealing with depression is hard and a nonstop battle. What I mean by that is even if you are getting professional help and taking medications to fight your depression, you may still have long periods of everything being okay and you being able to function normally. Then, the next thing you know you are sunken down low again and having the thoughts of harming yourself. Depressed people have different ways that they think of hurting themselves. For example, someone may be thinking of suicide, while another make think of cutting their wrist. Another person may be thinking of burning themselves, while another person may self-medicate with drugs. There may be many times where you will never know if they do these things because they can wear long clothing or do the activities in places where they feel no one will look. For example, I have a friend that would cut their wrists, and between wearing long sleeves and a lot of bracelets, no one would ever know unless you pay attention to the small details.

People may not realize it, but a lot of times when people are being mean and rude to you, they themselves could be dealing with depression. Their way of dealing with it is making sure someone else feels worse than they do, and that usually involves name calling or telling you nothing that you do is good enough. However, the problem with this is that many people do not realize with so many people going through depression. You may not always know how deep that being rude or mean will cause a person to sink. Also, with a person dealing with depression and being mean and rude to others, it only shows that you can be mean and rude for the moment to feel a sense of happiness for like a split second. Then you may find yourself returning to the sadness you had before you were mean or rude to someone around you.

Some people end up with depression because they are bullied and made fun of because of what they wear or for who they want to date. But one of the main thing's kids must deal with now is coming out about them liking the same sex and wondering what is going to happen to them when most people find out. Usually this leads to the child trying to take their life because of all the hate comments they receive from peers around them. With them not be able to be their self it tends to be harder for them to go through life. They will be depressed because they feel like they are less human and alone and a bad person.

Then there are some kids who get depressed because their parents do not love them when they need it the most. For example, when a parent has you clean the whole house by yourself and the stepparent does not have any roles in the house and lay around, they get down and feel they are not loved. Parents must realize that you must be careful how you treat your child compared to someone who is now in the picture. If you do not see the person that you are helping out in anyway and you have your child doing everything than that makes them feel more like a maid or servant than part of the family with love.

Depression sucks when you feel abandon and you feel like you should not exist because it feels like the whole world is against you. People must realize everyone needs love, without love people tend to become cruel and broken hearted. For example, if you do not give a child a childhood that will let them be just a kid, they become depressed because they see other kids around them that are having fun and they are not. Also making a child do things like them worrying about not having enough money to pay the bills and them having to get a job at a young age to help the family out can be very depressing to them. There are even the cases where some parents show favoritism to one child and not the other. The one child that is not the favorite will be depressed and feel like they were not meant to be on this earth are part of the family. Which in turns when they get older if they have kids while thinking of what happen to them as a child, that it must be how their children should be raised.

Depression can also come from a kid telling their parent information about their life and the parent goes and discuss it with other people. This creates a situation where the child will start keeping things to themselves verses talking about them with the fear of other people finding out. It will not only make them depressed, but they will start to lose trust with people that are around them in the fear of them telling all their business and not having someone to confide in.

Children can become depressed if you are a parent or adult talking about other people they love and care about. It makes the hurt because they know the person or people, they are talking about are caring or loving. And then if the child hears it and then goes repeat it back to the person they were talking about the child will get in trouble, and then the parent wants to fuss and yell at the kid for only repeating what they heard come out of their parents mouth.

Orphans become depressed especially around the holidays because where most kids are getting toys and love a lot of these kids are not getting anything. Most of the kids only wish to be a family with someone who genuinely cares for them. They are sad because they hate that the people that made them did not want them. It could also be the fact that their parents died, and no other family members wanted to take them in. With them they may never feel like they are whole are that they should exist. A lot of times if they find one good person that sticks by them, they turn out to be like family to them. With the kids being depressed they tend to get into a lot of trouble because they feel alone in this big world. Once a lot of these kids get bigger, they tend to be what most people would call loners because they are not used of having people to help them.

Something a parent should not do is tell your child that they cannot follow their dreams and that it is out of reach for them. For example, never tell your child that they will not make it to be famous. You never know what can happen for them and this will sadden your child. But at the same time let them know what could happen as far as they may not succeed but have a backup plan so that if their dream does not work out they have something else to fall back on. Encourage your kids every day because you never know what they are going through when they are not around you and around all these people that may be strangers to you. Just like you never know that they are depressed because at school when they eat lunch they may be all alone or have no friends at all and be a total out cast. They could come home and go to their room and cry themselves to sleep at night because they are feeling unloved. Which in turn this behavior can end up with the child trying to kill themselves or them acting out to get attention from people that they feel like are ignoring them.

Depression can come from the fact of people telling them they need change every day. In other words, telling them not to be themselves but act like someone you can be proud of. The thing is if they are meant to change or want to change, they will. But unless they are doing something that is illegal or that can harm them let them know that they are perfect the way that they are. Because now a days so many people whether male or female needs to know that just because they may not look like the people they see in books or on television that they are beautiful or handsome in their own ways. Because a child will get depressed dealing with not looking like the cool kids and so many of the kids making fun of the way they look or dress.

Depressed people can find it even harder to deal with their depression when you have family members that think they know what you are going through, or they do not realize that you are being bullied by someone in your own family. This can range from a parent, sibling, aunt, uncle, or even an in law. When you have depression, I think the best way for these people to understand is to communicate with them. However, sometimes when you have another person that is not willing to communicate, it becomes extremely hard to cope with. Just like if you know a person is dealing with depression and you are having a disagreement with them, let them cool down, especially if they ask for some space. Pressing the issue can make them want to harm themselves. Not allowing a depressed person or any person for that matter to have space can be a mistake by them rushing out of the house because you would not let them have the space to think. In this case, just imagine if they get behind the wheel of a car and are not thinking straight. It could end up with them being involved in a car crash that could take theirs, or someone else's life. Some things are better to talk about after you both calm down, because talking when both parties are heated can tear people apart including relationships.

      Just like anxiety, depression can cause a person to not eat or drink. When some people are depressed, not eating can be their way of dealing with the pain. The person may drink things such as soda, sports drinks, or water to fill up on. While you have this type of depressed person, you will also get the person who will eat and drink everything to find comfort in those things. Then you will have the depressed person who will try to get drunk or high every moment of everyday. What depressed people who partake in these behaviors do not realize is that the only reason they must do this every moment of everyday is to keep that numbing feeling going in your system. I have personally noticed when I am depressed, I keep myself active whether it is working out, or doing a hobby I love. The activities will brighten my mood and bring me out of my depression to a certain extent.

      Having depression can make you feel like you are being smothered and not being able to find a way to get air into your lungs. With me, when I am depressed, it feels like my head is completely confused and that my world is spinning at a hyper speed. Depression for me can feel like I have been hit by an eighteen-wheeler truck. It is like it hit me, and then it backs up on me a few times. It does not kill me, but it leaves me badly hurting to the point where I cannot get any kind of medical care for it. It also feels like no one can see the damage that has happened, and that people just think that you are faking. They feel like you are not being real, and that you are crazy to the degree of not being stable. When you know someone dealing with depression, please try not to make them feel like they are crazy and need a straight jacket. I know with me that if I get on social media sites, I often see a lot of people lying about the things they have or seeing a lot of my true friends post about how sad they are. The thing is looking at fake things and sad things can also make depression in you come out stronger than ever. I noticed that once I limited social media and started focusing more on myself, I figured out things that will help clear my mind.

      What a lot of depressed people fail to realize is that when you do things that you enjoy, you tend to be in a better mood. When you are in a better mood, you tend to have less thoughts of harming yourself. A friend once told me when you are thinking of harming yourself, try to think of it as being selfish to the people who absolutely love you and that you love back. I know while being depressed I hate hearing things like this, because I want people to feel and understand the pain that I am going through and just like a kid, give me the okay to feel like this. But from this person who fights with depression, it is better a lot of times to have at least one good friend who will tell you the truth as long as they're not brutal with it.

      Remember if you need to know how to start a conversation with someone that you think has depression, there are hot lines and websites that you can use to be able to start these conversations. Remember that it is always better to have these kinds of conversations than not to and end up with a person trying to take their own life. If you truly care about the person and they especially turn out to have depression, then you will have either them talking to you about why they're depressed, and you can help them to get help. You can also ask and hope that they will tell you what the problem is. Either way, it is a winning situation because you are helping a person learn to cope and deal for another day.

      You never know what a person has been through for them to have depression. In my case, much of my depression comes from the fact of losing my mother at the age of nineteen. Seeing her take her last breath is a moment that will be with me for the rest of my life. The depression aspect came into play when instead of dealing with my mom's death, I pushed all my feelings down and tried to keep moving. It was so bad that I was even in my mind pretending that the only reason that I was not seeing her was because she was in the hospital, and that I had to continue to work to make money. It felt like it got so busy to the point where I just never had time to go see her, and that is how I dealt with it. It was not till I went to a counselor that I realized my depression was growing from me not dealing with the grief. I noticed the more I started to talk about it, I realized one of the main reasons I was depressed because I felt like I was starting to lose the sound of her voice, as well as a lot of memories about her.

  Sometimes people get depressed about some things that most people just learn to fix and move forward from. For example, a person might get depressed because they gain weight and may not have the figure that they have had since they were younger. To most people, the most obvious thing to do is to exercise and change your diet, but to a depressed person, they take it as not being confident and more. Before you laugh at a person with depression over this, you first must ask yourself if this person has someone who is talking about them maintaining a certain weight to look a certain way. For example, imagine if a woman gets married to a guy and he is especially into her for her looks. What happens when she gives birth and does not know how to balance the life that was going on before the baby and add exercise in with the fact of waking up multiple times throughout the night for the baby? I mean I have heard of some women who have given men kids in which he tries to teach his children to disrespect their mom. I have heard of these types of guys even making her do things like mow the lawn or will not let her speak to male neighbors because he is thinking that she is flirting with them. However, the true thing that caused her depression in this way is the fact that they had a swimming pool, and if she wore a bikini, he thought she was fat and would tell her to go on a diet. Which in this case would make her feel less about herself, and unloved for the way she was.

  People get depressed in relationships where their partner or spouse is controlling or abusing them. The people in these relationships usually never know that the person is this controlling until they get further into the relationships. Because the person is now in love with the other person in the relationship, no matter how much they are mean and controlling towards them, they hang in there because they feel like they will come around eventually. This can depress them, and the only way they can come out of being depressed is by letting go. Usually when they let go of the person, they are often still depressed because they feel they lost someone that they believe love them. This kind of depression can happen within family member relationships. With the family relationships, it is usually the fact that they use a person that they love, especially when that person will do anything to make sure they have what they need. Giving your last to people that do not appreciate you can aid in causing depression. This happens because a lot of times when you have those kind of family members, it depresses you that you are not able to get the same amount you put into loving your family.

  People fail to realize that usually when a kid is getting bullied, they tend to get depressed and afraid to go to school. Usually when a kid is in love with school and are happy to see their friends, then suddenly that changes, there usually is a problem. You can usually tell if they are depressed by them changing from doing things like snacking a lot or not enough, to their grades falling in school. This especially applies if they are a straight A student. There might even be kids who try to get someone to drop them in the middle of the road so a car can hit them. With the child having depression, they may even try to harm themselves with household items such as knives or fire. So, if you have kids, make sure to pay attention to your children and how their moods and body language are. If you cannot get them to talk to you, always try to get them some professional help. Remember that with a kid, you would rather catch the problem early and get help than to let it continuously grow till it gets worse.

Some children develop depression over their parent or parents constantly telling them that they must stay focus on school with not a lot of fun. When parents do not let their children interact with other kids their age and have fun, it can cause them to have depression. I mean if all you let your child do for fun is math, English, or some type of study, this can cause them to be sad and unhappy. When they get depression from this, a lot of times as the child gets older, they will be depressed and start to rebel to get to experience some fun in their lives. Remember just like you needed fun when you were younger a child needs it, and you do not want them to grow up to fast and being depressed at that. Adults also forget that things for children now a days is not as easy as we had it.

Adults will get depression sometimes from losing their job or feeling like they can never get their dream job and they are stuck. Adults are depressed because to make sure they have all they need in life they sometimes must be okay with staying at the job they are apt to make ends meet. There is also the thing of sometimes no matter how much you try to get another job, it is like you are stuck in the job you are working, which in turn makes a person depressed. When it comes to jobs so many people try to please their parents by doing the job that they want you to do, when it is whatever makes you happy. Being stuck in a job that is dead end is the worst, because you know you cannot move up. Adults also get depressed because they are sometimes not given the opportunity to show the skills they have and so they will promote someone they are friends with over what a person can do. It is sad to think that now a days to be able to get into the right top positions it is all about who you know, and not what degree or skills you have. Adults get depressed when it is time to retire from a job and they cannot continue to work in their field. When people are like this it means a few things that they may not have family to go home to or that they really enjoyed being a part of something or they absolutely loved the job.

Military people tend to get depressed from being away from their families for weeks at a time. Some even get depressed because they must miss special events of their families to work. Normal people never realize how much stuff we take for granted, like most people in the military miss their kids first steps or first words. Soldiers tend to get depressed when they must go to war and leave their family behind and not know whether they will make it back to see them. Which when you think about most spouses must sit at home or try to work and keep their mind off whether their family will come home the same way they left. But soldiers will also get depressed when they get out and try to go back to civilian life, it now feels so different for them and that they feel out of place.

Blaming yourself is a way that can also cause you a lot of depression in your life. Like one of the things that I blame myself for is my best friend's death. Now before anyone jump to conclusions, no I did not kill him. It was the fact of me video calling and talking to him and the conversation ended, and I tried to call back and I could not get through. I kept trying for a couple of days till finally I went on his Facebook page and realized that he had died from an accidental mishap not long after getting off the call with me. Because I was one of the last people to talk to him, I figured if I stayed on the call longer that he would still be alive. And the blaming got worse when a family member of my friend blamed me too. But I had to figure out that him dying was out of my control and that no matter what it was just his time to leave this earth. I had to realize that by blaming myself I was only hurting my mental health and that I had to be okay with him passing, which does not make it any better. I finally forgave myself and started grieving him more and gave up the idea of it being my fault. When a close person dies in a crazy way, just remember it is not your fault and that they would rather you only think of the good times with them.

        Depression can even come from being in the military and being able to help people in natural disasters. Military people may get depression seeing all these people around them going through these traumatic experiences. For example if a person in the military is deployed to a disaster area like when hurricanes hit and flood an area or destroy it, they are the first ones in to try to rescue people who need to get to safety. With me going through having to be rescued by the military, sometimes we forget that while yes, we are suffering and scared, we forget that soldiers will put themselves in harm's way to save you. That can make them depressed thinking about what if their families were in this same predicament how they would feel. As well as them putting themselves in harm's way can make them depressed because they do not know if they will make it out alive to see their families, and to be able to do a lot of things they like to do that are especially hobbies. So, when you are sitting there and upset at not having material things, there are others who are fighting to make sure that they can help others and keep themselves alive.

        People also forget that some people are depressed because of what they do not have that they may need. Meaning a person that has no legs might be sad if they see all their friends and family members walking around and they do not know what it would be like to walk around without help. Then you have those that will be extremely depressed if they have some kind of accident and they lose their legs they will be upset and embarrassed because they cannot use their legs and are called crippled by so many people. These same people may be down because they feel like less of a person for not having their limbs working the way society make it seems normal. They will get depressed because they go places and people will stare at them like they are broken. So, when you see people that are not considered society normal, remember not to stare and be friendly they are still just as human as everyone around them.

        Depression can also come from people that have a loved one serving in the military and they must wonder every day if they will come home in one piece. When it comes to military families a lot of times one person is stuck at home with the kids trying to make sure they are okay and do not forget the loved one that is so far away for months at a time and the kids cannot see them. The person that is in the military must miss their kids miserably because they miss a lot of the kid's firsts. People only think of the person that is serving in the military as the only one that can get depressed when they never realized that basically the family of this person is also serving with them, because they a part for so long. Usually you have the other parent stepping in to take care of the kids or other family members because both parents are in the military on leave.

        Depression can come to some children who lose their parents and have to live all their lives without their parents especially if they knew and loved them, it is a difficult task for them to move having to live with another family member. They will get depressed with the fact of never getting to hug or hear their parents voices again. Depression creeps ever more in when they feel like they are forgetting what their parents smell like as well as how their voices use to sound. I know for a fact that the feeling of not remembering your loved ones hurts, and even with just the thought of it make me want to cry and wish that I could hear my loved ones voices again. I feel like a horrible person because I cannot remember all these things, which makes me feel like I was never worthy of them. And not feeling worthy of yourself turn all those feelings into depression because you become sad and feel worthless.

        With having depression, it causes a lot of people to want to sleep, which in turn we tend to not want to do anything or be around anyone. Sleep and depression will sometimes keep a person from pursuing their dreams and even give up working or doing their favorite hobbies from just wanting to be asleep. Some people with depression will start to neglect their hygiene and even go as far as not to eat, because the mental pain they feel, feels worse than anything else that is going on around them. With me when I get overwhelmed it is like my mind shuts down and I cannot focus on anything and I become lazy and do not want to do anything. It can also make the work that you must do come out super sloppy and wrong till you end up jobless because your work is horrible. I know with me not getting enough sleep and having depression is the worst combination because it makes you sensitive to simple mistakes or a person that normally annoys you but you are okay, turns into you being super annoyed and frustrated with them.

  Depression sometimes will make you push away all friends and family because you feel like if you let people get close, they will only leave. And if you fall in love with them that you feel so broken that no one will ever want to be with you. Depression makes you feel so broken that you just feel like that no matter what you will never be fixed, and you cannot think about dating. When it comes to dating and being broken you feel that no one will ever date or marry you because you are broken from depression. When you feel like you are broken from depression the first thing you should do is find out why you feel broken. Once you figure out why you feel broken then try to figure out ways to fix it.

  Depression is something that can turn your blue sky's to only black sky's, basically mean you might be this happy person all the time and one day wake up and you are gloomy. I mean everyone has these types of days, but it is the kind that never leaves, and you feel like the world is moving at a fast pace and your world is slowing down. It may seem like all your friends and family are always happy and have good things happening to them and you are stuck in a world with none of these things happening. It even gets to the point of you looking at a happy movie and with no way to cheer up to laugh at the show that you are watching.

  Depression can happen because of some of life decisions that we make. For example, if a person has a heart and abort a child that they know they cannot afford to pay for a child and give them security. I mean when you do things that are crazy like that it comes up and you sometime regret the things you did. When you think of these things you a lot of times become depressed and regret the fact of doing whatever it is. Being depressed some people may decide that is too much to bear. The worst part is that you figure out that you can forgive yourself for what you have done, but then later turn around and blame yourself for the same thing.

  Holidays can make people depressed for more than one reason. Two of the main holidays that most people go through that make them depressed is Christmas and Valentine's Day. Most people get depressed on these days because you tend to miss family members or long for a partner in life seeing people around you have all kind of fun. The other thing that will get people in their feelings if you lose a loved one around these times, it becomes hard to celebrate. Depression can come because you have no one to spend your holidays with like family or friends. You never know who is depressed and is hiding behind their smile to make it seem like they are okay, and that they will be okay spending the holiday alone, when in reality they are screaming help me by inviting me to come over. Holidays can sometimes be ruined by wanting to get through them quickly to forget about the loved ones we have lost at that time. It hurts to go through holidays knowing that your favorite loved one is not there and it reminds them of how bad they are missing them. Sometimes it makes us want to go back into the pass because you want to relive the days when they were here.

Depression is also brought on by losing a lot of pictures and memories of someone that you genuinely care about. As well as if you see pictures of people that have hurt you from your pass all those memories will come flowing back. If you have the problem of bad memories coming back from pictures that means you have not let go of those hurt feelings and forgive them, I did not mean forget, it means forgive them so that you can move forward and give yourself peace in your heart. When you lose pictures and things that a person gave you that you were truly close with dies away those things becomes priceless to you. When you lose this stuff sometimes you can replace the items, but it will not hold the same value as it would have been coming from the loved one that is now deceased. You may also lose interest in something that a loved got you started in because it hurts too much to think of the person every time you do it. For example before my mom died I had always wanted to learn to play piano, so she enrolled me in piano lessons I was taking them still when she became very ill, when she passed away I could not find the courage to go on with the lessons when I knew I could not come and play the songs I learned for her so I quit. Now that I am trying to better my mental health I am looking into finding a piano teacher and getting back into playing piano, because I know my mom would want me to continue to play the piano and become very happy making music. With when you are depressed over something like this, I am sure the person that you loved would want you to continue with life and not stop living.

   Depression is something that some people think that if they hang out with a person that has it, they will end up with it. People must realize that depression can be a cause of a chemical imbalance in your brain. But most of the time depression comes from within a person who is going through hardships or thinks too much about the what ifs or what I should have done. The other reason is people try to control any and everything around them when that is impossible. People forget a lot of times that no matter how much we want to be in control of everything in our lives or family lives it is impossible. The only thing you can be in control of is the decision that you make in your life and how you live but outside of that there is no way to control other things or beings around you.

   Depression can come from falling in love with someone and putting them on a pedestal and then they break up with you, this is usually a way a person becomes depressed and afraid. You should never get super attached to a person to the point that if they leave you, you tend to have a meltdown, and become very depressed. When you get in this state of depression it just means that we put all our trust in a person. In this case you need to take better care of yourself and your mental health than to worry about who wants to walk out of your life. I had to come to the realization that not everyone is meant to stay in your life. It even came a time in my life where every relationship that I had gotten into and it failed I thought that it was my fault. I figured that they did not work because I am too aggressive or that I did so many things wrong, but I could not figure out why. Which in turn with my depression I started to realize that I was actually pushing people away so I would not get hurt or that I would not get rejected or somehow screw up a relationship and hurt anyone else as well.

   Depression is not something that you can go without being treated for because I found out the hard way that a lot of times it gets worse the more you go through hardships. The more I let myself be depressed the more I thought that my life did not matter to anyone ant that no one genuinely cared about me. I even went to the point of I thought I was invisible, and that if I stood in front of people that no one was looking at me but through me. There was even a time when I thought that people only wanted to help me out with things because I was like a charity case to them. I felt that when people would tell me I was beautiful or sweet or a kind person, I figured they were trying to be nice and that they really did not mean it. I even felt that I was an ugly duckling and that I was a very evil person, while I am out there helping others get out of their struggles and to help them towards their dreams. I even felt that I needed attention from people to be happy when reality all I needed was to love myself and find ways to make myself happy. Without treating my depression, it was like my world was spinning out of control and there was no way I could get it to stop. I know that to get where I am now, I had to go through a lot of different medications, counseling, and seeing a psychiatrist that got me to get my depression under control.

  While there are a lot of single mothers out there, many may be ok raising their child or children alone, while others are having a hard time. What I mean by this is think about all the women who got married and got pregnant and then suddenly, she loses her husband; this also go for single dads. I mean you never know that the persons spouse could have died in battle, a disease, or just died. And remember some people may not have others to lean on during these times. It may be the person having to trust a total stranger with their child just to be able to go to work or have an adult break. I mean the fact of trying to make sure you have everything covered from what the kids needs to what they want.

  Some women be depressed when they find out that they will never get to have a child of their own. Whether they cannot have a child because of medical reasons or they cannot find the right guy to have the child with. To a woman this may make her feel less than a woman, because it has been thought of as a society thing if you cannot bring a child into this world. So being that she is ashamed this may sadden her a great deal as well. She will get depressed every time someone ask her when they are going to have a baby, and she knows that she cannot have one unless she gets a surrogate or adopt a child.

  People may not realize that when some women have a baby they go into a deep depression. It might even get to the point of where she does not want to have anything to do with her own child. It also does not mean she does not love her child. But if she shows this while in the hospital usually the nurses and doctors will help her by either giving medications or letting her talk to an in-house therapist. When the new mom goes home hopefully, she has someone who is by her side for a little while to help because she can end up being really depressed to the point, she may try to harm the baby. When it comes to dads if you are left with your child and cannot deal with the child crying, let someone know call someone to help or someone you trust because otherwise there could be some serious problems.

  You also have some adult children who may end up being depressed because their parents may not like the job they chose because to them they do not make a lot of money. Parents must realize that just because your child does not make the money you want them to, if they are happy doing what they are doing, you should be happy for them. If I had a child, I would rather them be happy doing what they are doing, because you never know whatever they are doing could lead to something that is extraordinary. Give the child room to grow and make mistakes because the more you smother them the more likely that you will not get what you want them to do out of them. Then on top of that you may send your child spiraling down with depression because they are not accomplishing what their parents want them to accomplish.

  There are also those kids who end up with depression because they have a parent that is in a profession that is very embarrassing. For example, if you have a child who wants to make something out of their lives, but people only see how their parent is out in the streets selling drugs, that might sadden the child. A child can also be depressed from having to live in their parent's shadows. For example, if the child has a parent that is doing really big things in life, they expect the child to be able to follow in their parent's footsteps. The child may be depressed because they are really wanting to do something else with their life. Parents need to let their kids know that it is okay not to follow in their footsteps and to be better than them, as well as make sure they find something that they will be happy doing for the rest of their life.

      No matter what depression is a real mental illness that we need to start to address more and not pretend that this is not a problem. The more we let this mental illness go on without making help readily available or ignoring depression the more people we will have trying to take their lives or a child's. As well as we need to let people know that it is not something to be embarrassed by, and that we will not treat them differently. And for people that do not have to deal with this mental illness, do not judge the people around you and make them feel less than human, because if you were in their shoes you would want someone to do the same for you.

      One of the top things to remember is that if you want to help keep your loved one around, try to get them help. There are different ways you can do this. If you feel like someone is going through depression and you genuinely care, find ways to talk them into getting professional help. You never know who you help by finding ways towards a better mental health and may be keeping them alive to see another day. If you know someone is changing rapidly and things really feel weird, try to have a conversation with them. If you cannot get through to them, try to find someone that will. Always find a way to get to the bottom of things. Depression take a lot of lives these days.

PTSD

Post traumatic stress disorder (PTSD) is something that I also deal with. Before I get more into that, I want to let it be known that I was not in the military. What a lot of people do not understand that anyone can have PTSD. You can get PTSD by going through something that is very traumatic for you. I got my PTSD from two very traumatic experiences. The first was a car wreck that I was in, and the second was from Hurricane Harvey. You might ask how a car wreck could be so traumatic? Well, when you happen to be in a small car and see a huge SUV truck coming towards your car at an angle as you are blowing the horn, and all you see is you jumping the curb of a gas station and hoping not to hit the gas pumps, it can lead to trauma.

Since the car wreck happened, when I drive now, I am paranoid that the cars on the side of me are going to hit me from the side. Now when I see a person driving crazy, I let them pass me, or I will pass them to make sure that I am safe and out of their way. I even tried to get through this by going through the same route; meaning I followed most of my steps from when the wreck happened. I even made it a point to drive in the same lane to prove that if I go that direction and did the same things, having an accident would not happen again. Even though I still have that fear and it scares me to death to drive knowing what happened, I also know that I cannot stop driving forever because I must get to work and other places. I cannot speak for anyone else, but I know that I hate waiting after work to be picked up.

With Hurricane Harvey, that was super scary because just as I got ready to get in the bed at midnight after knowing the people across the street already had water in their homes, water started to seep under the walls and doors into the house. I mean the first thoughts I had were this cannot be real, and then to hurry and pack a bag with clothes and medications to make sure I have the things I need. I could not leave my house by my vehicle, so I had to wait for either people in rescue boats to come through to get us. Being rescued by the boat would mean that more water would be pushed into the house. So, with no more power and the house filled with water at least three feet high, along with seeing your stuff floating around through the house is a weird experience. So basically, I had to wait till daylight when I was rescued by a military helicopter. They had to connect me to a harness, and the military personnel attached themselves to me as the helicopter hovered over me. Inside the helicopter, the other military personnel unstrapped me, and got me into the seat and buckled me in.

So, from the hurricane experience, every time I hear a helicopter in the sky, I have a flashback to the storm. I must breathe deep breaths and try to bring my mind back to the present. I must remind myself that with them being in the sky, they are doing practice runs to make sure if a bad hurricane happens again, they will be ready. I also must remind myself that every time that it rains hard that it does not mean that it will flood to the point that it did during the hurricane. I try to calm down and not have an anxiety attack and make things worse. I hate when I hear about hurricanes being in the water close to where I stay. My anxiety levels begin to rise, and I will start to try to watch the storms every move when I should focus on my work. There are a lot of times I must try to focus hard on my job and worry about the storm when I get off. With the storms in the water, I usually do not sleep well at night. I will toss and turn throughout the whole night.

Recently, I had to evacuate for Hurricane Laura because the path of the storm was headed directly for my city. I remember the night before leaving, I had a bad anxiety attack to the point of where I took my anxiety medications and started having flashbacks from when Hurricane Harvey hit. I had visions once again of being stuck standing in water. When you are stuck standing in water, you do not know when you are going to get to dry land to be able to get dry. Factor in that I was hoping that I would not get stuck in the water to where my feet cannot touch the ground. To put it in a thought that explains the feeling it felt like being able to breathe after holding your breath under water after falling into a pond, and someone is finally able to save you or you are able to get to the top to get to the air.

    So, if I am going through these things think about our military people who go to war to keep our country safe. I mean when they have flashbacks you never know what their eyes have seen in war and what they have a flashback about. If I could put my mind to think of what might cause them to have flashbacks, I would think of things like them seeing their fellow comrades being shot right in the front of them and not being able to save them for the fact of trying to keep themselves alive and keep us free. Some people in the military have flashbacks from when they lose a limb, I am sure they have nightmares about what they could have done differently to have saved their limbs. They may also have flashbacks from hearing gunfire and bombing all day and night and not know whether their location will be discovered. One of the major things that normal people do not realize is that people in the military may not get a lot of sleep during war, because they never know when they are being invaded, so they do not sleep much because they are scared for their lives. People in the military have all kinds of flashbacks and still try to lead normal lives. Just think what these poor people have gone through that normal people will never hear stories about, because a lot of them or to graphic and horrific to anyone that has not seen it, as well as a lot of times when they join the branches they are sworn to keep everything that they see behind the lines to themselves. That is why when I see them, I make sure to go out of my way to thank them because they went through or are going through so much so I can have my freedom.

    Most people do not realize that even people who work in our prison systems tend to end up with flashbacks. It come from dealing with rude inmates, that thinks they are the big and bad one in the prison so they start fights with another who has the same way of thinking in which the prison workers have to get involved and pull them apart and keep others from joining in. Prison workers a lot of times end up stopping riots from the prisoners, which takes a lot of force and authority. In these riots a lot of the prison workers get trampled and hurt, and they must worry about not getting killed in being trampled. So prison workers may have flashbacks of what they have been through of being trampled and it might even scare them when they need to go around big crowds that are not family, because they may think that a fight will break out and they will get trampled or hurt again and they cannot do what they do at work.

    Another thing that people may have flashbacks about are the fact that they have gotten molested, it does not matter whether it is a family member, family friend, or a stranger. Many people go through this and have flashbacks for lifetime which in the long run will cause them many health problems. I mean you never know to what extreme a person was molested and what they were told to try to keep them from telling on the person that did this to them. A lot of people go through it and have flashbacks but will not tell anyone because they are scared to get the person that done it in trouble, as well as most of them are embarrassed about how people will look at them after they tell. Many people have flashbacks about what happen but will not get help for being ashamed or embarrassed. So, these people also have flashbacks because they become older and no one helped them even after they revealed what has happen to them. Some of these people have flashbacks for more than one reason, it is because it was a family member and when the person got in trouble it tore the family apart and a lot of the family blame you for it. Some people even get flashbacks from watching movies that have explicit scenes in them and may get upset and people may not understand why they are that way. People that have been through this may have flashbacks from seeing pictures of themselves from the time of the event it brings up what has happened to them. They may also have flashbacks especially if it was a family member and they run across pictures at another family members home of them.

   Flashbacks may happen when the person was raped in public by an unknown stranger, or even someone you think that is a friend, work with or go to school with. What people do not realize is that when a person start closing themselves off from meeting new people and being around people that have been around but are in maybe the same workspace of school, they are terrified of the same thing that has happen before to happen again. When a person must go through this other people must realize that it is now hard from them to trust other people because this is a very traumatic experience. To explain this better it is like going to eat at the same restaurant and ordering the same thing as time goes on it seems to taste different, so you stop eating there because you want the old taste back, but you know you cannot. When a person has this traumatic experience happen it is extremely hard for them to trust again because they have flashbacks of their privacy being taken from them. Just think of someone stealing something that is valuable to you not money but a memoir or something you know you can never get again for you, from a stranger, co-worker, classmate, or teacher.

   People sometimes end up with PTSD from seeing a love one die or get badly hurt to the point they cannot do the things they use to do with you. In my case it was when I found out my mom had cancer and they could do nothing more than give her medications to keep her comfortable from pain, and when they gave her pain medications they made her hallucinate that she had something crawling all over her. I flashbacks a lot of times when I pass the hospital that she was in, and wondering if there was something, I could have done to help her feel better. Now if for any reason I need to go to the hospital, I am scared that they are going to give me the wrong dose of medications and I will die. And I had another flashback when I went to the hospital for my knee because it was so swollen all I could wear was leggings because it was swollen bigger than a baseball, to say they are a hospital they stuck me seven times without being able to get nothing but blood out when they said it was filled with fluid. So the next day I had to go to see a doctor that specializes in bones and joints to get the fluid drawn out of my knee, and while waiting I became very scared and nervous because I did not know if it was going to end like it did in the hospital. The other ways people might have flashbacks if they see their loved one getting taken away in a body bag. If you truly think about it even though they may not be breathing when they get put in one, you still want it to be open with the hopes of them starting to breathe all of a sudden. Every time I think of my mom being brought out of our house in a black body bag I tear up and want to go sit in a corner somewhere away from the world. Just like if a family member of yours fell and injured themselves badly in a way that would not hurt most, it would make a person have a flashback every time they see someone doing that action.

   There are women out there that have PTSD because they may have been through a process where they were pregnant, and they run into another female or male and lose their kid. What I mean is the woman may have her child forcibly taken from her body, after carrying the baby almost to term. Then after the baby is forcibly taken the mom will never see it again because the other person took the child to raise as their own. For the mother she may have flashbacks every time she passes another child. They may have a flashback every time they pass the place where her baby was taken from her. If the mother in this case decides to try to have another baby while fighting to find her first, she may quit her job and all activities till she has her baby. The only place she may go is the doctor and back home, and hope and pray all the way home that she does not have what happen the first time happen again.

   There are women who struggle because they lost a child. Whether they lost their child while they are carrying them. Even if they lose their child right after having them. There are the ones that lost their child in a tragedy. So, with the mother that loses her child while carrying it will have flashbacks if her and her husband try again. She will become scared that she will get to the same month as the last child and lose this one. With her having this going on she may shut herself down from everyone around her till her baby is born.

   Children can even have PTSD from being bullied at school constantly and feeling alone and no one can help them, they will feel like it will only make things worse. There are children that are going without eating because people are taking their lunch money or even taking their plates off the table and throwing their food away. So, a lot of times these kids are going through the rest of their day hungry and unfocused. A lot of time if a kid is extra super hungry than they normally are they are more than likely not getting to eat at school. They might be dealing with a person giving them wedgies or beating them up without leaving really a mark. A lot of times when a kid is scared to go to school are asked to change schools is because they are being bullied. They might end up with flashbacks if they are playing around with cousins and they pretend they are going to give them a wedgie they may get upset at the cousin and not want to play anymore.

   Remember to keep at the struggle of having flashbacks and that they are only a horrible memory. That you are now safe, and you have people that love you surrounding you. Never be afraid to reach out for medical professional help to keep you feeling like yourself most of the time.

ALL THREE TOGETHER

If you have all three anxiety, depression, and PTSD your life tends to be very crazy and hectic. When you start out you do not realize what is going on with you so you feel like every bad thing in the world that should be happening to everyone, is only happening to you. When you are hearing certain sounds that remind you of something bad you have been through, and when something really upset you till you cannot breathe and your heart races, and lastly you wish you did not exist. When you have all this going at once is like putting an animal in another habitat that they really do not belong in. In other words, it is like being confusing and while you hate yourself, you sometimes want to be able to help others and make sure they do not feel as confused and horrible as yourself. With me it was easier to help others because it was like it helped me forget about all my problems and emotions and focus on someone else.

I realized I needed to get help to sort through everything I was going through. At first it was not easy to talk to my doctor about me having depression because I was embarrassed. Then the doctor told me I needed to sit down with a counselor to see what was causing all this depression. My first session with the therapist I thought it would be hard to tell a stranger my problems and my business, but on the first day I broke down in tears over my mom's passing. The more that I started to go the less my life started to feel confused. I found out that a lot of my reasoning for feeling the way I do is because instead of letting my anger or any feelings out, I was actually taking them in and pushing them down instead of letting them out. Which means that I now try to speak my mind and try to move forward.

With a person dealing with all these, one thing that they should try to do first is love yourself, because no one will love you as much as you love yourself. When you start to love yourself first you will always be happier and what others do will not matter. The more you care about yourself and go through hard times, the more you will see who your real friends are as well as who in your family will be there for you. The more you take care of yourself the more you will see that you do not need others to give you approval about who you are the way you are supposed to dress or feel about yourself.

Dealing with all three of these together and seeing how hard it is to make it through a day, and then I stop and see how far I have come, and I am proud of myself. I remember days when I thought of driving myself off a really tall bridge, to trying to mix medications to end it all, and my attitude towards people who were trying to help me through this type of things was horrible. When they would try to give me simple advice like breathe and I would get mad and tell them that they did not understand anything I was going through. I also thought that no one ever wanted to be around me or that they truly really cared about me. When it came to me liking guys it was like the ones I wanted, I scared them away by my thinking I needed them to complete me and my life would go back to normal. With the guys that I liked I would go from being sweet to seeming like I was needy and clingy. I felt the only time I was at peace was when I was sleep or away from everybody and just by myself. Then it came down to me not being able to sleep at night, all I would do is toss and turn with thoughts of how to end it all, or how the people around hated me or thought I was a completely horrible person. I mean all my friends really tried different tactics to get me to feel better, and it was like it would not work, I went as far as to drink cups of alcohol and then take the pills that I was given to try to help with depression, anxiety, and PTSD, which everyone knows you are not supposed to mix alcohol and medications. With me drinking the alcohol it only made my depression worse at the time, making me think harder about my insecurities.

It took me to make some changes in my life for me to become happier and that is something that is not easy at all. It took my friends talking to me and showing me motivational things and how things in their lives were the same as mine sometimes, and how they deal with them. They made me realize that I was not crazy to get help with my problems, and that there are plenty of people that deal with at least one of the things I am still battling with. Once I started trying to get out of my negative world, and tried to come to the positive side, especially after I started realizing that my friends really cared and I was hurting them with me telling them that I did not want to exist or I should not exist. I knew then that I had to do something, as well as seeing some of my younger family members dealing with depression and anxiety, I knew then that I had to be a better role model for them, and stop being so self-centered around me. I knew I had to figure out a way of thinking, but I had to enlist the help of my friends. I had them help me by not letting me talk to negative about myself and them reassuring me that I was loved and cared for. It was plenty of times when I know I drove them crazy by saying that they did not love me or care for me, and them telling me over and over that they did. Even now if I tell them that I think I am fat they tell me I am not, and if I am unhappy about my weight to exercise and eat healthy.

The counselor I went to told me to try to journal and see if that help as a way for me to get my feelings and emotions out, and as time went on to look back to see how much I had changed. I did this for a little bit but I got scared people would get a hold of it and read them, which I got one with a code and tried again and I just could not do it. But thanks to a friend I was shown that I could create a blog and write about different topics, which turned out to be a great idea because I always wanted to write a book. A lot of times I thought that I would fail at the blog or many other things that I wanted to do but thanks to my friends they would not let me give up on my dreams. I have also decided that I will be there for them and support their dreams as best as I can. I realized that I also have young kids looking up to me and the things I do, so I must live right and be better for them. Because I want them to grow up and have a better outlook on life, so they do not think that being an adult is all bad and that adults are never happy. And I also know that with me being around kids that have a touch of depression, it is better to show them that they can work through it and not to give up, because they will always have the fact that I am still here fighting for life and making it more of a happier one.

With me having all three things I have started to realize what things trigger my anxiety, depression, and PTSD, and I am trying to find ways around them. I know one thing that many people do not realize that can affect their moods and these types of mental illnesses, it is music. When all a person listens to is upbeat music talking about killing, drugs, and explicit material, it will start to have a negative effect on the way you start thinking. It also comes down to certain beats and tones they can have a negative impact, because think if you have slow sulky beats it can make you become sad, even though you may have started your day in a happy mood. I know personally for me once I stopped listening to a lot of the music on the radio every day and started adding more of inspirational or motivational speeches to listen to I have been in a better mood, as well as I have been able to function without thinking negatively. With me making this small change it is like the time now flies super-fast when I am working or at home, while at the same time taking time to enjoy the simple things around me. I feel more confident in my decisions I make and while my plate feels full, I do not feel so overwhelmed.

I have also noticed that I do not feel like I am stuck in life anymore, I feel like there is a whole world out there waiting for me. I feel like even though I have not found the right job for me yet that I am going in the right direction even though things may not always go my way. I think that way now because I have realize that when I think positive I feel like my day goes better that way, verses me thinking of all the negative things that can go wrong in my day. I feel like the more I think of my day being great and I confirm it in my heart that it will be. I started realizing that I was letting people and everything about certain things where I work get to me when it should be that I move on and not let it control me. I truly have learned that there are very few things in this world that should make you upset and make you want to end your life. I found out sometimes people will try to make you end your life so they do not have to deal with you but it is better to make them look like a mean person or like they cannot be beat up or messed with.

    If you are like me do not give up the fight of fighting all three illness because then everything and everyone that said you would fail wins. I know you have it in you to keep fighting for a happy productive life.

Summary

      Everyone should really take time to notice the people and problems around them if not in the world at least in your community. I am quite sure that there are people who could just use a listening ear. We all know that it does not cost much to lend a listening ear, yes it cost time. I would rather give up my time then to lose a person in the community because no one had time to listen. I also know that just listening sometimes is not enough to fix the problem, but just like smiling at someone can brighten their day or change it, it is the same with listening to what they are going through.

      Also remember that you never know what a person is going through so make fun of no one and treat everyone how you like to be treated. If you say the wrong things to someone it could end up with them not living. Sometimes all a person need is someone to be kind and show they care at least a little. Be the change you want to see in this world, by helping someone fight through these mental illnesses. Just because you deal with them and are fighting through it does not mean someone else is able to deal with them and fight. Just because you have the illnesses does not mean you cannot be someone's light to them fighting through and making it out on the other side.

      Anxiety is real and if you deal with it remember to try to breathe through it and find your happy place as best as you can. Just remember there is someone else that may be going through the same things and they deal with anxiety as well. Also remember that just because someone does not have the same ways of having an anxiety attack it does not mean the person does not have it. Learn the triggers of your anxiety and find ways to stop them ahead of time with either medication or natural herbs. May you be able to fight anxiety and be to the point of functioning every day without the scare of having one. The breathing exercise I do is taking a deep breath in through your nose while counting to ten, and release through your mouth slowly counting to ten. Breathing like this usually helps me get through an anxiety attack and stopping it early. While the guided imagery helps get my mind off things while breathing. Remember you got this, and this will pass.

      So when you get mad at someone and think that just because someone has a smile on their face constantly, it does not mean that they have no problems it just mean they try to deal with them and move on. Then you never know this person may be smiling in front of people but really dying on the inside. Sometimes it is better to treat people the way you want to be treated because you may never truly know what they are going through. Meaning that even though they smile, or they may tell you a little about them behind the scenes you may never know the true full story. The other thing people need to realize is that just because a person has a smile does not mean that they are happy, people sometimes use their smiles to hide their pain. Always remember that anyone can be depressed no matter the age, and you never know what a person is going through.

      PTSD is a hard thing to get through and is not really a way to get over it because the flashbacks are real and painful. As scary as things are, I just want you to know to keep your head up and know that you can get through these episodes no matter how scary they are. I know there will be days that will get the best of you, but with me these are days that I make myself fight the hardest and make it out on the other side. Just remember when it comes to PTSD, that the biggest key to it is fighting through the flashbacks and coming out on the other side of the flashback a stronger person. No matter how hard it may seem to me you are a strong person and that shows you that you are stronger than you think. So just give it your all and do not let the flashbacks stop you from living life and achieving your dreams.

      I hope after reading this book you learn to think about your words and actions towards another human being. I hope that everyone checks in on your loved ones with all the turmoil that is going on in this world now a days. Remember that with everything that is going on make sure you truly check in on the people of the world that you know, they may need a helping hand and may be holding it in because of embarrassment or the thought of making the situation worse. Hopefully if one of your friends or family members are going through one of these things, you will jump in and try to help or show them that you are there for them with support in some form. The more we show one another that we care and are there for one another, the better this world will be. I mean if we can help one less person go through these and stop people from trying to end their lives. People can volunteer to help our veterans and military people by being there for them. People always forget sometimes people only need another person to take time with them or listen to what they have to say. Remember just to KEEP FIGHTING!

www.ingramcontent.com/pod-product-compliance
Lightning Source LLC
Chambersburg PA
CBHW080818220526
45466CB00011BB/3607